The Mediterranean Diet For Beginners

An Easy And Understandable Guide To Discover The Secrets To Lose Weight With A Meal Plan And Simple, Easy And Healthy Mediterranean Diet Recipes

Lacy Holland

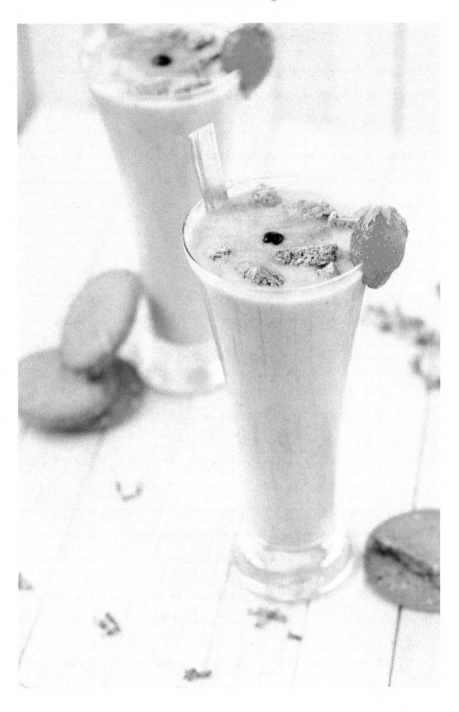

Table of Contents

VEGETABLES AND SOUP 44

MEAT RECIPES 60

FISH & SEAFOOD 70

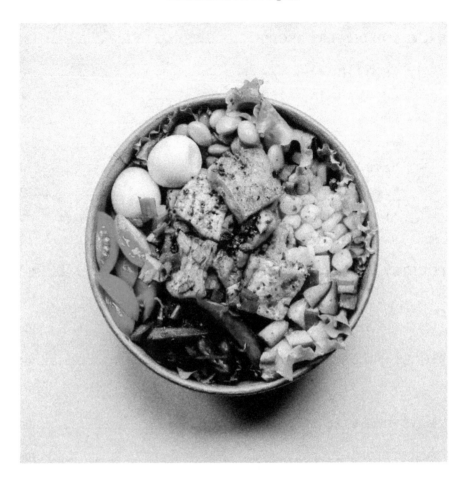

Introduction

The Mediterranean diet is based on the culinary habits of Mediterranean islanders such as the Romans and Greeks. Fruits, bread, wine, olive oil, nuts, and seafood were abundant in these regions' diets. Despite the presence of fatty foods in their diets, residents of this area appeared to live longer, healthier lives with less cardiovascular problems. In the 1950s, American scientist Ancel Keys discovered this phenomenon.

In the 1950s, Keys worked as an academic researcher at the University of Minnesota, where he studied healthy eating patterns and how to reverse America's cardiovascular health decline. In his study, he discovered that poor people in the Mediterranean region were healthier than the rich American population, which had recently seen an increase in coronary heart disease and obesity. In comparison to affluent New Yorkers, the Mediterranean lower class lived long into their 90s and remained physically active into their senior years. Keys and his team of scientists agreed to travel the globe in order to investigate the relationship between a region's diet and the wellbeing of its inhabitants. In 1957, he traveled to the United States, Italy, Holland, Greece, Japan, Finland, and Yugoslavia to study habits, nutrition, exercise, and diet.

According to Keys' study, people in the Mediterranean region had a longer lifespan and were more physically active than people in other parts of the world because of their dietary choices. Greeks, in particular, enjoyed a diet rich in good fats such as meat, nuts, olive oil, and fatty fish. Despite the high fat content of these foods, their cardiovascular health remained stable, with no signs of a heart attack or stroke. His research was used to help the United States develop its own dietary standards, and he was dubbed the "Father of Nutritional Science."

Further studies and clinical trials on the Mediterranean diet have been undertaken as a result of Keys' work, providing evidence for its health-improving properties. You can lose weight while also lowering your LDL "negative" cholesterol, lowering your blood pressure, and lowering and stabilizing your blood sugar levels. You will significantly reduce the risk of suffering from a heart attack, stroke, or premature death by reducing these symptoms of coronary heart disease.

It's important to remember that these improvements in someone's health cannot be accomplished exclusively by the Mediterranean diet. It can be determined by a host of other lifestyle factors such as genetics, physical activity, smoking, obesity, substance use, and so on. Incorporating physical activity into your life is an essential part of the Mediterranean diet. That's how the Mediterranean "diet" becomes a Mediterranean "lifestyle" that closely resembles the people of the region. Greece's citizens lead an active lifestyle, engaging in some kind of physical activity on a regular basis. Rolling, sailing, rowing, swimming, or hiking are all examples of physical activity that can be paired with a balanced plant-based diet to achieve positive health outcomes. Physical exercise in today's world could include a trip to the gym or even a simple walk around the street. It doesn't have to be strenuous; the main thing is to include some kind of physical activity in your day so that you can reap the full benefits of this diet.

The Benefits Of A Mediterranean Diet

The Mediterranean diet offers a number of health benefits that are not seen among people who consume that much red meat. The diet is associated with a lower risk of death from cancer, heart attacks as well as strokes, and even a lower number of deaths from Alzheimer's. There's also a list of other benefits such as a lower risk of high blood pressure, depression, and other chronic diseases and a better quality of life. If you ever wanted a taste of the good life, here are some of the top benefits of the Mediterranean diet.

Lower Risk Of Heart Disease

Unlike most people associated with the term "diet" with losing weight, this diet as stated earlier will help you live longer. Heart disease is one of the leading causes of death in the U.S. This diet simply helps you reduce some of the factors that lead to a heart attack. In the study done on British men, those who opted for the Mediterranean diet had a 41% lower risk of dying from a heart attack when compared to those who followed the more traditional high-fat diet such as the Atkins diet.

Lower Risk Of Stroke

It is not just the heart that benefits from the diet, but your brain too. People who consumed the Mediterranean diet regularly had a 22% lower risk of suffering an ischemic stroke than those who were following a high-fat diet. The study also found out that strokes caused by other factors such as bleeding tended to be less severe in people who ate vegetables and fish as the diet recommended. People who suffer strokes normally have a hard time recovering from it and the factors that lead to it need to be avoided.

Boost Immunity

You wouldn't know it, but your body's immune system is a strong part of your vulnerability to some of the diseases that plague you. This diet regulates the immune system and keeps the body strong and protected in the fight against infections.

Lower Risk of Cancers

Eating the right meals can ward off different types of cancer without having to resort to painful treatments or harsh pharmaceuticals. In the United States alone, death by cancer is the second leading cause of death. This diet is known for its cancer-fighting properties. The Mediterranean diet has been associated with lower risks of cancer in general. Not only does it help in killing various existing cancers but it also prevents cancer cells from forming in the first place. The Phytochemicals in fruits and vegetables found in this diet cover all of the cancer-fighting departments. The diet also has Omega 3 fatty acids which help fight inflammation, and even help prevent the spread of cancerous cells.

Lower Risk of Diabetes

The Med-diet or Mediterranean diet is the magic diet to go to in order to lower the risk of diabetes in both men and women. People who eat this type of diet not only reduce their risk of getting diabetes to begin with but they also boost protection. This diet keeps blood sugar levels under control and helps people avoid the need to get medication for the condition. People who eat this type of diet have also been shown to lower their risk of heart disease and stroke which can lead to diabetes.

Protection From Diabetes

People who have a diet that is rich in fruits and vegetables will have an easier time in keeping diabetes at bay. The diet for diabetes is similar to the Mediterranean diet. The diet helps people control their weight by eating healthy foods. These foods are rich in complex carbohydrates. The elimination of red meat and sugar from one's diet will also boost metabolism.

It is never too late to start a healthier diet. You can start at any time and change yourself into a healthier person. Start with small changes and make a beeline towards the Mediterranean diet. You will be surprised at how your body will change for the better. There is no need to suffer from diseases, complications, and even death just because you decided to overeat regularly. You can protect yourself by eating healthy. There is no need to be cruel to your body and compensate for the harm you did before.

Benefits Of The Mediterranean Diet For Women Over 50

Boosts Your Brain Health: Preserve memory and prevent cognitive decline by following the Mediterranean diet that will limit processed foods, refined bread, and red meats. Have a glass of wine versus hard liquor.

Improves Poor Eyesight: Older individuals suffer from poor eyesight, but in many cases, the Mediterranean diet has provided notable improvement. An Australian Center for Eye Research discovered that the individuals who consumed a minimum of 100 ml (0.42 cup) of olive oil weekly were almost 50% less likely to develop macular degeneration versus those who ate less than one ml each week.

The Risk of Alzheimer's disease is reduced: In 2018, the journal Neurology studied 70 brain scans of individuals who had no signs of dementia at the onset. They followed the eating patterns in a two-year study resulting in individuals who were on the Med diet had a lesser increase of the depots and reduced energy use - potentially signaling risk for Alzheimer's.

Helps Lessen the Risk of Some Types of Cancer: According to the results of a group study, the diet is associated with a lessened risk of stomach cancer (gastric adenocarcinoma).

Decreases Risks for Type 2 Diabetes: It can help stabilize blood sugar while protecting against type 2 diabetes with its low-carb elements. The Med diet maintains a richness in fiber, which will digest slowly while preventing variances in your blood sugar. It also can help you maintain a healthier weight, which is another trigger for diabetes.

Suggests Improvement for Those with Parkinson's disease: By consuming foods on the Mediterranean diet, you add high levels of antioxidants that can prevent your body from undergoing oxidative stress, which is a damaging process that will attack your cells. The menu plan can reduce your risk factors in half.

Higher Energy Levels: Diet is one of the most important things that will help you in the process of losing weight to make yourself fit. Having a healthy diet, even if it is as simple as eating healthy foods, will definitely give your body a sense of energy.

List of Typical Foods of the DM

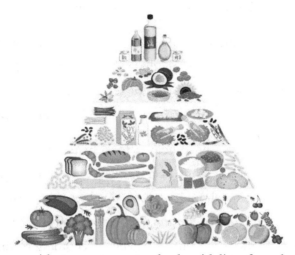

The food pyramid serves as a standard guideline for what a healthy, well-balanced diet should look like. It was created by the United States Department of Agriculture (USDA) so individuals could better follow and understand recommended food servings. The USDA food pyramid offered Americans an easy-to-follow template of what they should eat daily.

This food pyramid has been under continual attack, and several other versions were released before the most well-known version was made public in the 1990s. Food companies criticized each of the previous versions, stating it would cause the general public to stop buying their products (Roycor, A., and Roycor, A., 2017). It seems as though the food pyramid that was created did not take the health of the people in the United States into consideration but was more of a marketing stunt for food companies.

At the bottom of the USDA pyramid, you will find the grains food group with the recommendation of 6 to 11 servings a day. This group includes bread, pasta, rice, and cereals. Above the grains are the fruits and vegetables. Fruits have a recommendation of 2 to 4 servings a day, while these vegetables recommend 3 to 6 servings.

Next up on the pyramid is a line that divides up the dairy and meat food groups. Dairy is recommended to be consumed 2 to 3 times a day. The meat group, which includes red meats, poultry, fish, beans, eggs, and nuts, recommends that you eat 2 to 3 servings a day.

While this pyramid may have helped food manufacturers boost sales, there is a great deal of controversy around it. It has not specified which types of grains should be consumed or that healthy fats and unhealthy fats are grouped are the first discrepancies. The other is the daily recommendations are out of balance. According to this pyramid, your diet should consist mostly of grains.

Recently, a newer design of the pyramid is being used. Instead of a pyramid, it uses a plate to show individuals how much each food group should fill their plates at each meal. While there is a noticeable difference in portion size, vegetables seem to fill more of the plate than the other food groups. Fats are often completely left out of the diagram.

To combat the original USDA food pyramid, the Mediterranean food pyramid came about. The Mediterranean diet pyramid was created with the Harvard School of Public Health and the World Health Organization (WHO) (Oldway's Mediterranean Diet Pyramid, n.d.). It showed foods displayed in the same pyramid formation. Still, it didn't include daily recommendations for all food groups and further divided groups in affordances to their health benefits. The foods at the bottom of the list should be consumed daily. The foods in the middle of the pyramid should be consumed a few times a week. And foods at the top of the pyramid should be consumed every month.

According to the Mediterranean diet pyramid, extra virgin olive oil and other healthy fats like nuts and seeds, along with whole grains, fruits, vegetables, legumes, and beans, sit at the bottom of the pyramid. Above this large section, you will find the fish and seafood group. Next is poultry, eggs, cheese, and nonfat dairy. At the very top of the pyramid is the red meat and sweets group. There are some significant differences between the USDA food pyramid and the Mediterranean diet pyramid.

First, the USDA grouped all meat on the pyramid. There is no distinction between whether you should eat more red meat or fish for better overall health.

The Mediterranean diet clearly emphasized fruits, vegetables, and healthy fats to be consumed daily. It also made physical activities and connecting with others a priority. No other diet took into consideration the importance of these last two factors. While everyone suggests exercising for losing weight, it is rarely suggested as part of a diet plan to live a long healthy life.

It is argued that the Mediterranean diet is not an ideal diet for most people around the world to adapt to. As you continue to read, you will learn just how simple it is to begin transitioning to a Mediterranean diet. You will see that all the food groups included in the Mediterranean diet are easily available no matter where you live.

Foods to Eat

The table below has a comprehensive list of foods that you should be eating on the Mediterranean diet.

The foods are divided into two categories:

Foods You Should Eat Liberally: You can eat these foods every day- as much as you want because they hold most of the diet's nutritional benefits.

Foods You Should Eat in Moderation: Although the Mediterranean diet is not restrictive- you are pretty much allowed to eat anything you want, but there are some foods that you are advised to eat in moderation.

These foods are generally healthy but may contain some elements that, when consumed in excess, may have negative effects on the body.

	Foods You Should Eat Liberally	Foods You Should Eat in Moderation
Grains	<ul><li>Oatmeal (Steel-cut or Old-fashioned)</li><li>Whole grain bread (made with whole wheat flour)</li><li>Quinoa</li><li>Bulgur Wheat</li><li>Farro</li></ul>	<ul><li>All bran cereal</li><li>Pasta</li><li>Polenta</li><li>Couscous</li><li>Whole grain crackers</li></ul>
Proteins	<ul><li>Beans</li><li>Chickpeas</li><li>Tempeh</li><li>Lentils</li><li>Tofu</li></ul>	<ul><li>Eggs</li><li>Chicken</li><li>Seafood</li><li>Fish</li></ul>
Oils and Fats	<ul><li>Extra-virgin olive oil</li><li>Olives</li><li>Avocado Oil</li><li>Avocado</li></ul>	<ul><li>Canola Oil</li></ul>

| Fruits and Veggies | <ul><li>Zucchini</li><li>Dark Greens</li><li>Egg Plant</li><li>Artichokes</li><li>Bell Peppers</li><li>Blackberries</li><li>Peaches</li><li>Blueberries</li><li>Cherries</li><li>Raspberries</li><li>Apricots</li><li>Strawberries</li><li>Potatoes</li><li>Sweet potatoes</li><li>All root vegetables</li><li>Starchy Veggies</li></ul> | |

Nuts and Seeds		<ul><li>Almonds</li><li>Pistachios</li><li>Walnuts</li><li>Cashew Nuts</li><li>Pecans</li><li>Macadamia Nuts</li><li>Brazil Nuts</li><li>Hazel Nuts</li><li>Peanuts</li></ul>
Dairy		<ul><li>Goat Cheese</li><li>Plain Greek Yogurt</li><li>Feta Cheese</li><li>Brie</li><li>Plain Ricotta</li><li>Milk</li><li>Cottage Cheese</li></ul>

Sweeteners		• Honey • Brown sugar (Small amounts of sugar added in coffee or tea)
Sauces and Condiments	• Pesto • Balsamic Vinegar • Tomato Sauce (sugar-free)	• Tzatzaki • Aioli • Tahini
Drinks	• Tea • Coffee • Water	• Red Wine • Alcohol
Herbs and Spices	• All dried herbs and spices • Garlic • All fresh herbs and spices	

Food to Avoid

The below list contains a couple of foods that you need to avoid when on a Mediterranean diet completely. This is because they are unhealthy and when you eat them, you will be unable to experience the benefits of a Mediterranean diet. These foods include;

Processed meat- you should avoid processed meats like bacon, sausage and hot dogs because they are high in saturated fats, which are unhealthy.

Refined oils - stay away from unhealthy oils like cottonseed oil, vegetable oil and soybean oil.

Saturated or Trans-fats - good example of these fats include butter and margarine.

Highly processed foods – avoid all highly processed foods. By this, I mean all the foods that are packaged. This can be packaged crisp, nuts, wheat etc. Some of these foods are marked and labeled low fat but are actually quite high in sugar.

Refined grains - avoid refined grains like refined pasta, white bread, cereals, bagels etc

Added sugar- foods, which contain added sugar like sodas, chocolates, candy and ice cream should be completely avoided. If you have a sweet tooth, you can substitute products with added sugar with natural sweeteners.

Now that you know what to eat and what not to eat when on the Mediterranean diet you are now ready to learn how you can adopt the diet.

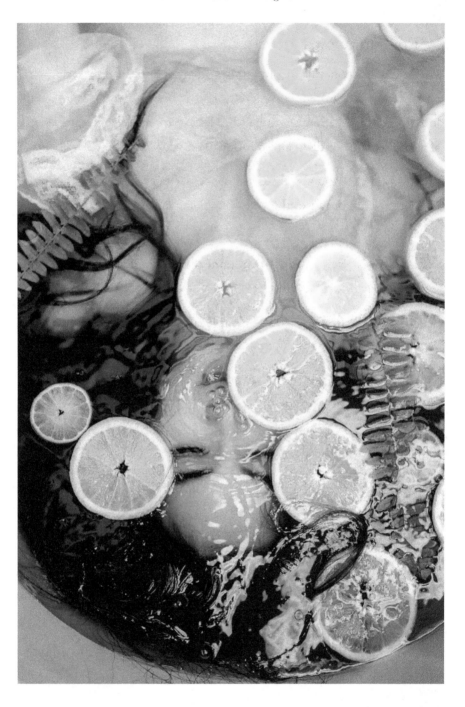

Common Mistakes

Researchers have researched a number of diets and nutritional philosophies for various health benefits over the years. The Mediterranean diet also comes out on top when it comes to overall benefits, as it tends to lower the risk of type 2 diabetes, heart disease, and other chronic illnesses.

The Mediterranean diet refers to the common dietary habits of Mediterranean countries such as the coasts of Spain, France, Italy, Greece, Turkey, Egypt, and Libya. Fruits, vegetables, whole grains, beans, nuts, seeds, fish, seafood, and healthy fats like olive oil are consumed in greater quantities in these regions, while red meat, refined foods, and added sugars are consumed in lesser amounts.

However, following a Mediterranean diet does not guarantee that you will be healthier. This heart-healthy diet, like any other eating pattern, necessitates some forethought to avoid making mistakes.

While perfection should never be the target and balance is essential, be wary of the following popular blunders that could jeopardize your Mediterranean diet:

1. Excessive use of oil

Yeah, it is possible to get too much of a good thing. Although the Mediterranean diet is renowned for its acceptance of olive oil—and healthy fats in general—you may want to refrain from drizzling oil over your entire meal.

Consider this: The ideal amount of fat per day is around 30% of your total calories, so one or two tablespoons per meal should suffice.

2. Drinking too much alcohol

Wine is a common part of the Mediterranean diet, but just a glass with dinner, not a half-bottle (sorry). In small quantities, alcohol does have potential health benefits, including a possible beneficial effect on cholesterol levels.

However, you can get all of the benefits of alcohol from other (less risky) sources, such as fruits and vegetables. According to the American Heart Association, drinking too much alcohol can cause health problems including alcohol use disorder, hypertension, stroke, and breast cancer.

Drink water with most of your meals to stay on board with the Mediterranean diet.

3. Speeding through meals

Many people mistakenly believe that the Mediterranean diet is all about the food, but it is really more of a culture or way of life. The Mediterranean diet emphasizes eating slowly, mindfully, and sometimes with pleasure.

That's because eating slowly helps you feel more comfortable with your meal, and studies have shown that people who eat slowly consume less calories.

To put it another way, eating on the go, at your desk, or in front of the television cannot be the best option. Instead, find a peaceful, distraction-free place and eat with others whenever possible. Try putting your fork down in bites or eating with chopsticks to slow things down.

Breakfast Recipes

1. Berry Breakfast Smoothie

Preparation Time: 3 minutes

Cooking Time: 0 minute

Servings: 2

Ingredients:

- 1/2 cup vanilla low-fat Greek yogurt

- 1/4 cup low-fat milk

- 1/2 cup blueberries or strawberries

- 6 to 8 ice cubes

Directions:

1. Place the Greek yogurt, milk, and berries in a blender and blend until the berries are liquefied. Mix in ice cubes and blend on high. Serve immediately.

Nutrition:

98 calories 10g fats 7g protein

2. Mediterranean Omelet

Preparation Time: 7 minutes Cooking Time: 12 minutes

Servings: 2

Ingredients:

- 2 teaspoons extra-virgin olive oil

- 1 garlic clove 1/2 red bell pepper

- 1/2 yellow bell pepper 1/4 cup thinly sliced red onion

- 2 tablespoons chopped fresh basil

- 2 tablespoons chopped fresh parsley

- 1/2 teaspoon salt 1/2 teaspoon black pepper

- 4 large eggs, beaten

Directions:

1. In a big, heavy skillet, cook 1 teaspoon of the olive oil over medium heat. Add the garlic, peppers, and onion to the pan and sauté, stirring frequently, for 5 minutes.

2. Add the basil, parsley, salt, and pepper, increase the heat to medium-high, and sauté for 2 minutes. Slide the vegetable mixture onto a plate and return the pan to the heat.

3. Heat the remaining 1 teaspoon olive oil in the same pan and pour in the beaten eggs, tilting the pan to coat evenly. Cook the eggs just until the edges are bubbly and all but the center is dry, 3 to 5 minutes.

4. Either flip the omelet or use a spatula to turn it over.

5. Spoon the vegetable mixture onto one-half of the omelet and use a spatula to fold the empty side over the top. Slide the omelet onto a platter or cutting board.

6. To serve, cut the omelet in half and garnish with fresh parsley.

Nutrition:

197 calories

18g fats

6g protein

3. Hearty Berry Breakfast Oats

Preparation Time: 11 minutes Cooking Time: 2 minutes Servings: 2

Ingredients:

- 11/2 cups whole-grain rolled oats

- 3/4 cup fresh blueberries, raspberries, or blackberries, or a combination

- 2 teaspoons honey

- 2 tablespoons walnut pieces

Directions:

1. Prepare the whole-grain oats according to the package directions and divide between 2 deep bowls.

2. In a small microwave-safe bowl, heat the berries and honey for 30 seconds. Top each bowl of oatmeal with the fruit mixture. Sprinkle the walnuts over the fruit and serve hot.

Nutrition:

204 calories 17g fat 4g protein

4. Garden Scramble

Preparation Time: 9 minutes

Cooking Time: 13 minutes

Servings: 2

Ingredients:

- 1 teaspoon extra-virgin olive oil

- 1/2 cup diced yellow squash

- 1/2 cup diced green bell pepper

- 1/4 cup diced sweet white onion

- 6 cherry tomatoes, halved

- 1 tablespoon chopped fresh basil

- 1 tablespoon chopped fresh parsley

- 1/2 teaspoon salt

- 1/4 teaspoon freshly ground black pepper

- 8 large eggs, beaten

Directions:

1. In a large nonstick skillet, cook olive oil over medium heat. Add the squash, pepper, and onion and sauté for 4 minutes.

2. Add the tomatoes, basil, and parsley and season. Sauté for 1 minute, then pour the beaten eggs over the vegetables. Close and reduce the heat to low.

3. Cook for 6 minutes, making sure that the center is no longer runny.

4. To serve, slide the frittata onto a platter and cut into wedges.

Nutrition:

211 calories

17g fats

5g protein

Snacks and sandwiches Recipes

5. Cucumber Sandwich Bites

Preparation Time: 5 minutes   Cooking Time: 0 minute Servings: 2

Ingredients:

- 1 cucumber, sliced

- 8 slices whole wheat bread

- 2 tablespoons cream cheese, soft

- 1 tablespoon chives, chopped

- ¼ cup avocado, peeled, pitted and mashed

- 1 teaspoon mustard

- Salt and black pepper to the taste

Directions:

1. Spread the mashed avocado on each bread slice, also spread the rest of the ingredients except the cucumber slices.

2. Divide the cucumber slices on the bread slices, cut each slice in thirds, arrange on a platter and serve as an appetizer.

Nutrition:

187 Calories

12.4g Fat

4.5g Carbohydrates

8.2g Protein

6. Yogurt Dip

Preparation Time: 10 minutes   Cooking Time: 0 minute Servings: 2

Ingredients:

- 2 cups Greek yogurt

- 2 tablespoons pistachios, toasted and chopped

- A pinch of salt and white pepper 2 tablespoons mint, chopped

- 1 tablespoon Kalamata olives, pitted and chopped

- ¼ cup zaatar spice ¼ cup pomegranate seeds

- 1/3 cup olive oil

Directions:

1. Mix the yogurt with the pistachios and the rest of the ingredients, whisk well, divide into small cups and serve with pita chips on the side.

Nutrition:

294 Calories 18g Fat 2g Carbohydrates 10g Protein

7. Tomato Bruschetta

Preparation Time: 10 minutes Cooking Time: 10 minutes Servings: 2

Ingredients:

- 1 baguette, sliced

- 1/3 cup basil, chopped

- 6 tomatoes, cubed

- 2 garlic cloves, minced

- A pinch of salt and black pepper

- 1 teaspoon olive oil

- 1 tablespoon balsamic vinegar

- ½ teaspoon garlic powder Cooking spray

Directions:

1. Situate the baguette slices on a baking sheet lined with parchment paper, grease with cooking spray. Bake for 10 minutes at 400 degrees.

2. Combine the tomatoes with the basil and the remaining ingredients, toss well and leave aside for 10 minutes. Divide the tomato mix on each baguette slice, arrange them all on a platter and serve.

Nutrition:

162 Calories

4g Fat

29g Carbohydrates

4g Protein

8. Olives and Cheese Stuffed Tomatoes

Preparation Time: 10 minutes Cooking Time: 0 minute Servings: 2

Ingredients:

- 24 cherry tomatoes, top cut off and insides scooped out

- 2 tablespoons olive oil ¼ teaspoon red pepper flakes

- ½ cup feta cheese, crumbled 2 tablespoons black olive paste

- ¼ cup mint, torn

Directions:

1. In a bowl, mix the olives paste with the rest of the ingredients except the cherry tomatoes and whisk well. Stuff the cherry tomatoes with this mix, arrange them all on a platter and serve as an appetizer.

Nutrition:

136 Calories 8.6g Fat 5.6g Carbohydrates 5.1g Protein

Salad and Side Recipes

9. Balsamic Asparagus

Preparation Time: 10 minutes

Cooking Time: 15 minutes

Servings: 2

Ingredients:

- 3 tablespoons olive oil

- 3 garlic cloves

- 2 tablespoons shallot

- 2 teaspoons balsamic vinegar

- 1 and ½ pound asparagus

Directions:

1. Preheat pan with the oil over medium-high heat, add the garlic and the shallot and sauté for 3 minutes.

2. Add the rest of the ingredients, cook for 12 minutes more, divide between plates and serve.

Nutrition:

100 calories

10.5g fat

2.1g protein

10. Lime Cucumber Mix

Preparation Time: 10 minutes Cooking Time: 0 minute Servings: 2

Ingredients:

- 4 cucumbers ½ cup green bell pepper

- 1 yellow onion 1 chili pepper

- 1 garlic clove 1 teaspoon parsley

- 2 tablespoons lime juice

- 1 tablespoon dill

- 1 tablespoon olive oil

Directions:

1. Incorporate cucumber with the bell peppers and the rest of the ingredients, toss and serve as a side dish.

Nutrition:

123 calories 4.3g fat 2g protein

11. Walnuts Cucumber Mix

Preparation Time: 5 minutes Cooking Time: 0 minute Servings: 2

Ingredients:

- 2 cucumbers

- 1 tablespoon olive oil

- 1 red chili pepper

- 1 tablespoon lemon juice

- 3 tablespoons walnuts

- 1 tablespoon balsamic vinegar

- 1 teaspoon chives

Directions:

1. Mix cucumbers with the oil and the rest of the ingredients, toss and serve

Nutrition: 121 calories 2.3g fat 2.4g protein

12. Cheesy Beet Salad

Preparation Time: 10 minutes Cooking Time: 1 hour Servings: 2

Ingredients:

- 4 beets

- 3 tablespoons olive oil

- ¼ cup lime juice

- 8 slices goat cheese

- 1/3 cup walnuts

- 1 tablespoon chives

Directions:

1. In a roasting pan, combine the beets with the oil, salt and pepper, toss and bake at 400 degrees F for 1 hour.

2. Cool the beets down, transfer them to a bowl, add the rest of the ingredients, toss and serve as a side salad.

Nutrition:

156 calories 4.2g fat 4g protein

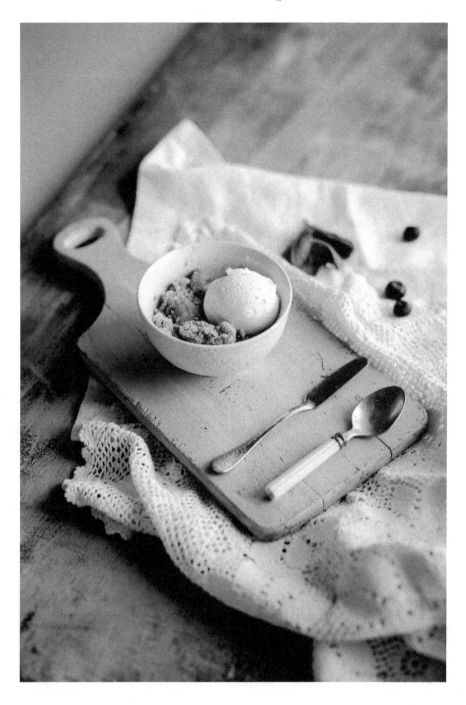

Vegetables and Soup

13. Cauliflower Steaks with Olive Citrus Sauce

Preparation Time: 15 minutes

Cooking Time: 30 minutes

Servings: 2

Ingredients:

- 2 large heads cauliflowers

- 1/3 cup extra-virgin olive oil

- ¼ teaspoon kosher salt

- 1/8 teaspoon black pepper

- Juice of 1 orange

- Zest of 1 orange

- ¼ cup black olives

- 1 tablespoon Dijon mustard

- 1 tablespoon red wine vinegar

- ½ teaspoon ground coriander

Directions:

1. Preheat the oven to 400°F. Prep baking sheet with parchment paper or foil.

2. Cut off the stem of the cauliflower so it will sit upright. Slice it vertically into four thick slabs. Situate cauliflower on the prepared baking sheet. Drizzle with the olive oil, salt, and black pepper. Bake for 31 minutes, turning over once.

3. In a medium bowl, combine the orange juice, orange zest, olives, mustard, vinegar, and coriander; mix well.

4. Serve at room temperature with the sauce.

Nutrition:

265 Calories

21g fat

5g Protein

14. Pistachio Mint Pesto Pasta

Preparation Time: 10 minutes

Cooking Time: 10 minutes

Servings: 2

Ingredients:

- 8 ounces whole-wheat pasta

- 1 cup fresh mint

- ½ cup fresh basil

- 1/3 cup unsalted pistachios, shelled

- 1 garlic clove, peeled

- ½ teaspoon kosher salt Juice of ½ lime

- 1/3 cup extra-virgin olive oil

Directions:

1. Cook the pasta following the package directions. Strain, reserving ½ cup of the pasta water, and set aside.

2. In a food processor, add the mint, basil, pistachios, garlic, salt, and lime juice. Process until the pistachios are coarsely ground. Add the olive oil in a slow, steady stream and process until incorporated.

3. In a large bowl, mix the pasta with the pistachio pesto; toss well to incorporate. If a thinner, saucier consistency is desired, add some of the reserved pasta water and toss well.

Nutrition:

420 Calories

3g fat

11g Protein

15. Burst Cherry Tomato Sauce with Angel Hair Pasta

Preparation Time: 10 minutes

Cooking Time: 20 minutes

Servings: 2

Ingredients:

- 8 ounces angel hair pasta

- 2 tablespoons extra-virgin olive oil

- 3 garlic cloves, minced

- 3 pints cherry tomatoes

- ½ teaspoon kosher salt

- ¼ teaspoon red pepper flakes

- ¾ cup fresh basil, chopped

- 1 tablespoon white balsamic vinegar (optional)

- ¼ cup grated Parmesan cheese (optional)

Directions:

1. Cook the pasta following the package directions. Drain and set aside.

2. Heat the olive oil in a skillet or large sauté pan over medium-high heat. Stir in garlic and sauté for 30 seconds. Mix in the tomatoes, salt, and red pepper flakes and cook, stirring occasionally, until the tomatoes burst, about 15 minutes.

3. Pull away from the heat then mix in the pasta and basil. Toss together well. (For out-of-season tomatoes, add the vinegar, if desired, and mix well.)

4. Serve with the grated Parmesan cheese, if desired.

Nutrition:

305 Calories

8g fat

11g Protein

16. Baked Tofu with Sun-Dried Tomatoes and Artichokes

Preparation Time: 30 minutes

Cooking Time: 30 minutes

Servings: 2

Ingredients:

- 1 (16-ounce) package extra-firm tofu

- 2 tablespoons extra-virgin olive oil, divided

- 2 tablespoons lemon juice, divided

- 1 tablespoon low-sodium soy sauce

- 1 onion, diced

- ½ teaspoon kosher salt

- 2 garlic cloves, minced

- 1 (14-ounce) can artichoke hearts, drained

- 8 sun-dried tomato halves packed in oil

- ¼ teaspoon freshly ground black pepper

- 1 tablespoon white wine vinegar

- Zest of 1 lemon

- ¼ cup fresh parsley, chopped

Directions:

1. Preheat the oven to 400°F. Prep baking sheet with foil or parchment paper.

2. Mix tofu, 1 tablespoon of the olive oil, 1 tablespoon of the lemon juice, and the soy sauce. Allow to sit and marinate for 15 to 30 minutes. Arrange the tofu in a single layer on the prepared baking sheet and bake for 20 minutes, turning once, until light golden brown.

3. Cook remaining 1 tablespoon olive oil in a sauté pan over medium heat. Cook onion and salt for6 minutes. Stir garlic and sauté for 30 seconds. Add the artichoke hearts, sun-dried tomatoes, and black pepper and sauté for 5 minutes. Add the white wine vinegar and the remaining 1 tablespoon lemon juice

and deglaze the pan, scraping up any brown bits. Pull away the pan from the heat and stir in the lemon zest and parsley. Gently mix in the baked tofu.

Nutrition:

230 Calories

14g fat

14g Protein

17. Baked Mediterranean Tempeh with Tomatoes and Garlic

Preparation Time: 25 minutes Cooking Time: 35 minutes

Servings: 2

Ingredients:

For tempeh

- 12 ounces tempeh

- ¼ cup white wine

- 2 tablespoons extra-virgin olive oil

- 2 tablespoons lemon juice

- Zest of 1 lemon

- ¼ teaspoon kosher salt

- ¼ teaspoon freshly ground black pepper

For tomatoes and garlic sauce

- 1 tablespoon extra-virgin olive oil

- 1 onion, diced

- 3 garlic cloves, minced

- 1 (14.5-ounce) can no-salt-added crushed tomatoes

- 1 beefsteak tomato, diced

- 1 dried bay leaf

- 1 teaspoon white wine vinegar

- 1 teaspoon lemon juice

- 1 teaspoon dried oregano

- 1 teaspoon dried thyme

- ¾ teaspoon kosher salt

- ¼ cup basil, cut into ribbons

Directions:

For tempeh

1. Place the tempeh in a medium saucepan. Add enough water to cover it by 1 to 2 inches. Bring to a boil over medium-high

heat, cover, and lower heat to a simmer. Cook for 10 to 15 minutes. Remove the tempeh, pat dry, cool, and cut into 1-inch cubes.

2. Incorporate white wine, olive oil, lemon juice, lemon zest, salt, and black pepper. Add the tempeh, cover the bowl, and put in the refrigerator for 4 hours, or up to overnight.

3. Preheat the oven to 375°F. Place the marinated tempeh and the marinade in a baking dish and cook for 15 minutes.

For tomatoes and garlic sauce

4. Cook olive oil in a large skillet over medium heat. Stir in onion and sauté until transparent, 3 to 5 minutes. Mix in garlic and sauté for 30 seconds. Add the crushed tomatoes, beefsteak tomato, bay leaf, vinegar, lemon juice, oregano, thyme, and salt. Mix well. Simmer for 15 minutes.

5. Add the baked tempeh to the tomato mixture and gently mix together. Garnish with the basil.

Nutrition:

330 Calories 20g fat 18g Protein

18. Roasted Portobello Mushrooms with Kale and Red Onion

Preparation Time: 30 minutes

Cooking Time: 30 minutes

Servings: 2

Ingredients

- ¼ cup white wine vinegar

- 3 tablespoons extra-virgin olive oil, divided

- ½ teaspoon honey

- ¾ teaspoon kosher salt, divided

- ¼ teaspoon freshly ground black pepper

- 4 (4 to 5 ounces) Portobello mushrooms, stems removed

- 1 red onion, julienned

- 2 garlic cloves, minced

- 1 (8-ounce) bunch kale, stemmed and chopped small

- ¼ teaspoon red pepper flakes

- ¼ cup grated Parmesan or Romano cheese

Directions:

1. Prep baking sheet with foil. In a medium bowl, whisk together the vinegar, 1½ tablespoons of the olive oil, honey, ¼ teaspoon of the salt, and the black pepper. Spread the mushrooms on the baking sheet and pour the marinade over them. Marinate for 15 to 30 minutes.

2. Meanwhile, preheat the oven to 400°F.

3. Bake the mushrooms for 20 minutes, turning over halfway through.

4. Heat the remaining 1½ tablespoons olive oil in a large skillet or ovenproof sauté pan over medium-high heat. Add the onion and the remaining ½ teaspoon salt and sauté until golden brown, 5 to 6 minutes. Stir in garlic and sauté for 30 seconds. Mix kale and red pepper flakes and sauté until the kale cooks down, about 5 minutes.

5. Remove the mushrooms from the oven and increase the temperature to broil.

6. Carefully pour the liquid from the baking sheet into the pan with the kale mixture; mix well.

7. Turn the mushrooms over so that the stem side is facing up. Spoon some of the kale mixture on top of each mushroom. Sprinkle 1 tablespoon Parmesan cheese on top of each.

8. Broil until golden brown, 3 to 4 minutes.

Nutrition:

200 Calories

13g fat

8g Protein

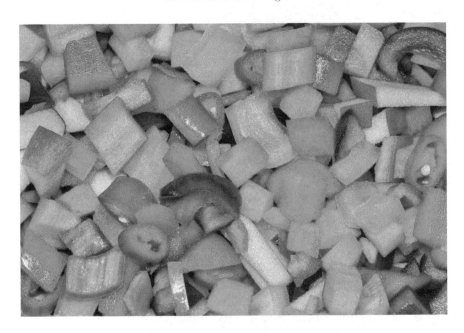

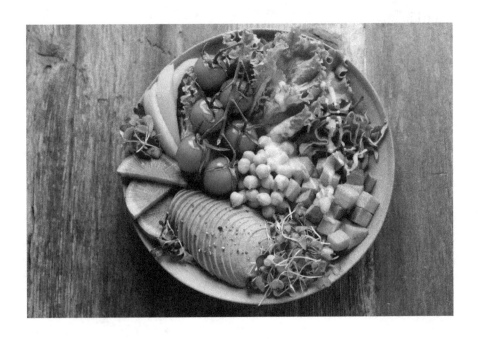

Meat Recipes

19. Mediterranean Pork Roast

Preparation Time: 10 minutes Cooking Time: 8 hours and 10 minutes

Servings: 2

Ingredients:

- 2 tablespoons Olive oil 2 pounds Pork roast

- ½ teaspoon Paprika cup Chicken broth

- 2 teaspoons Dried sage ½ tablespoon Garlic minced

- ¼ teaspoon Dried marjoram ¼ teaspoon Dried Rosemary

- 1 teaspoon Oregano ¼ teaspoon Dried thyme

- 1 teaspoon Basil ¼ teaspoon Kosher salt

Directions:

1. In a small bowl mix broth, oil, salt, and spices. In a skillet pour olive oil and bring to medium-high heat. Put the pork into it and roast until all sides become brown.

2. Take out the pork after cooking and poke the roast all over with a knife. Place the poked pork roast into a 6-quart crock pot. Now, pour the small bowl mixture liquid all over the roast.

3. Seal crock pot and cook on low for 8 hours. After cooking, remove it from the crock pot on to a cutting board and shred into pieces. Afterward, add the shredded pork back into the crockpot. Simmer it another 10 minutes. Serve along with feta cheese, pita bread, and tomatoes.

Nutrition:

361 Calories

10.4g Fat

0.7g Carbohydrates

43.8g Protein

20. Beef Pizza

Preparation Time: 20 minutes

Cooking Time: 50 minutes

Servings: 2

Ingredients:

For Crust:

- 3 cups all-purpose flour

- 1 tablespoon sugar

- 2¼ teaspoons active dry yeast

- 1 teaspoon salt

- 2 tablespoons olive oil

- 1 cup warm water

For Topping:

- 1-pound ground beef

- 1 medium onion, chopped

- 2 tablespoons tomato paste

- 1 tablespoon ground cumin

- Salt and ground black pepper, as required

- ¼ cup water

- 1 cup fresh spinach, chopped

- 8 ounces artichoke hearts, quartered

- 4 ounces fresh mushrooms, sliced

- 2 tomatoes, chopped

- 4 ounces feta cheese, crumbled

Directions:

For crust:

1. Mix the flour, sugar, yeast and salt with a stand mixer, using the dough hook. Add 2 tablespoons of the oil and warm water and knead until a smooth and elastic dough is formed.

2. Make a ball of the dough and set aside for about 15 minutes.

3. Situate the dough onto a lightly floured surface and roll into a circle. Situate the dough into a lightly, greased round pizza pan and gently, press to fit. Set aside for about 10-15 minutes. Coat the crust with some oil. Preheat the oven to 400 degrees F.

For topping:

4. Fry beef in a nonstick skillet over medium-high heat for about 4-5 minutes. Mix in the onion and cook for about 5 minutes, stirring frequently. Add the tomato paste, cumin, salt, black pepper and water and stir to combine.

5. Put heat to medium and cook for about 5-10 minutes. Remove from the heat and set aside. Place the beef mixture over the pizza crust and top with the spinach, followed by the artichokes, mushrooms, tomatoes, and Feta cheese.

6. Bake until the cheese is melted. Pullout from the oven and keep aside for about 3-5 minutes before slicing. Cut into desired sized slices and serve.

Nutrition: 309 Calories 8.7g Fat 3.7g Carbohydrates 3.3g Protein

21. Beef & Bulgur Meatballs

Preparation Time: 20 minutes

Cooking Time: 28 minutes

Servings: 2

Ingredients:

- ¾ cup uncooked bulgur

- 1-pound ground beef

- ¼ cup shallots, minced

- ¼ cup fresh parsley, minced

- ½ teaspoon ground allspice

- ½ teaspoon ground cumin

- ½ teaspoon ground cinnamon

- ¼ teaspoon red pepper flakes, crushed

- Salt, as required

- 1 tablespoon olive oil

Directions:

1. In a large bowl of the cold water, soak the bulgur for about 30 minutes. Drain the bulgur well and then, squeeze with your hands to remove the excess water. In a food processor, add the bulgur, beef, shallot, parsley, spices and salt and pulse until a smooth mixture is formed.

2. Situate the mixture into a bowl and refrigerate, covered for about 30 minutes. Remove from the refrigerator and make equal sized balls from the beef mixture. Using big nonstick skillet, heat up the oil over medium-high heat and cook the meatballs in 2 batches for about 13-14 minutes, flipping frequently. Serve warm.

Nutrition:

228 Calories

7.4g Fat 0.1g Carbohydrates

3.5g Protein

22. Balsamic Beef Dish

Preparation Time: 5 minutes

Cooking Time: 55 minutes

Servings: 2

Ingredients:

- 3 pounds chuck roast

- 3 cloves garlic, thinly sliced

- 1 tablespoon oil

- 1 teaspoon flavored vinegar

- ½ teaspoon pepper

- ½ teaspoon rosemary

- 1 tablespoon butter

- ½ teaspoon thyme

- ¼ cup balsamic vinegar

- 1 cup beef broth

Directions:

1. Slice the slits in the roast and stuff in garlic slices all over. Combine flavored vinegar, rosemary, pepper, thyme and rub the mixture over the roast. Select the pot on sauté mode and mix in oil, allow the oil to heat up. Cook both side of the roast.

2. Take it out and set aside. Stir in butter, broth, balsamic vinegar and deglaze the pot. Return the roast and close the lid, then cook on HIGH pressure for 40 minutes.

3. Perform a quick release. Serve!

Nutrition:

393 Calories

15g Fat

25g Carbohydrates

37g Protein

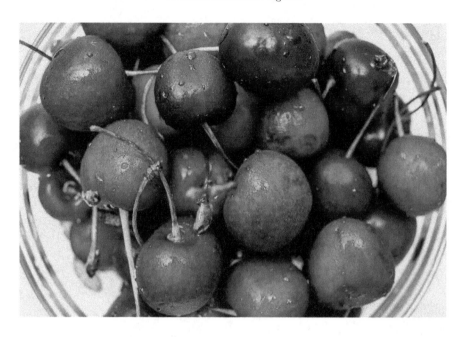

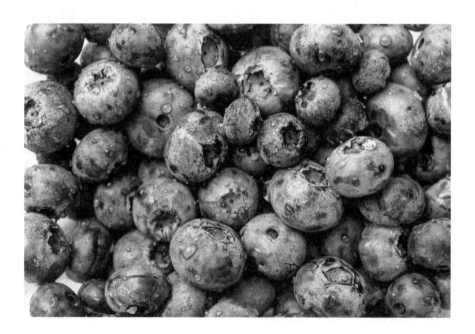

Fish & Seafood

23. Baked Balsamic Fish

Preparation Time: 10 minutes

Cooking Time: 10 minutes

Servings: 2

Ingredients:

- 1 tablespoon balsamic vinegar

- 2 ½ cups green beans

- 1-pint cherry or grape tomatoes

- 4 (4-ounce each) fish fillets, such as cod or tilapia

- 2 tablespoons olive oil

Directions:

1. Preheat an oven to 400 degrees. Grease two baking sheets with some olive oil or olive oil spray. Arrange 2 fish fillets on each

sheet. In a mixing bowl, pour olive oil and vinegar. Combine to mix well with each other.

2. Mix green beans and tomatoes. Combine to mix well with each other. Combine both mixtures well with each other. Add mixture equally over fish fillets. Bake for 6-8 minutes, until fish opaque and easy to flake. Serve warm.

Nutrition:

229 Calories

13g Fat

8g Carbohydrates

2.5g Protein

24. Cod-Mushroom Soup

Preparation Time: 10 minutes

Cooking Time: 20 minutes

Servings: 2

Ingredients:

- 2 tablespoons extra-virgin olive oil

- 2 garlic cloves, minced

- 1 can tomato

- 2 cups chopped onion

- ¾ teaspoon smoked paprika

- a (12-ounce) jar roasted red peppers

- 1/3 cup dry red wine

- ¼ teaspoon kosher or sea salt

- ¼ teaspoon black pepper

- 1 cup black olives

- 1 ½ pounds cod fillets, cut into 1-inch pieces

- 3 cups sliced mushrooms

Directions:

1. Get medium-large cooking pot, warm up oil over medium heat. Add onions and stir-cook for 4 minutes. Add garlic and smoked paprika; cook for 1 minute, stirring often. Add tomatoes with juice, roasted peppers, olives, wine, pepper, and salt; stir gently. Boil mixture. Add the cod and mushrooms; turn down heat to medium. Close and cook until the cod is easy to flake, stir in between. Serve warm.

Nutrition:

238 Calories

7g Fat

15g Carbohydrates

3.5g Protein

25. Mediterranean-Spiced Swordfish

Preparation Time: 10 minutes

Cooking Time: 15 minutes

Servings: 2

Ingredients:

- 4 (7 ounces each) swordfish steaks

- 1/2 teaspoon ground black pepper

- 12 cloves of garlic, peeled

- 3/4 teaspoon salt

- 1 1/2 teaspoon ground cumin

- 1 teaspoon paprika   1 teaspoon coriander

- 3 tablespoons lemon juice   1/3 cup olive oil

Directions:

1. Using food processor, incorporate all the ingredients except for swordfish. Seal the lid and blend to make a smooth

mixture. Pat dry fish steaks; coat equally with the prepared spice mixture.

2. Situate them over an aluminum foil, cover and refrigerator for 1 hour. Prep a griddle pan over high heat, cook oil. Put fish steaks; stir-cook for 5-6 minutes per side until cooked through and evenly browned. Serve warm.

Nutrition:

275 Calories

17g Fat

5g Carbohydrates

0.5g Protein

26. Anchovy-Parmesan Pasta

Preparation Time: 10 minutes

Cooking Time: 20 minutes

Servings: 2

Ingredients:

- 4 anchovy fillets, packed in olive oil

- ½ pound broccoli, cut into 1-inch florets

- 2 cloves garlic, sliced 1-pound whole-wheat penne

- 2 tablespoons olive oil

- ¼ cup Parmesan cheese, grated

- Salt and black pepper, to taste

- Red pepper flakes, to taste

Directions:

1. Cook pasta as directed over pack; drain and set aside. Take a medium saucepan or skillet, add oil. Heat over medium heat.

2. Add anchovies, broccoli, and garlic, and stir-cook until veggies turn tender for 4-5 minutes. Take off heat; mix in the pasta. Serve warm with Parmesan cheese, red pepper flakes, salt, and black pepper sprinkled on top.

Nutrition:

328 Calories

8g Fat

35g Carbohydrates

7g Protein

27. Garlic-Shrimp Pasta

Preparation Time: 10 minutes

Cooking Time: 15 minutes

Servings: 2

Ingredients:

- 1-pound shrimp, peeled and deveined

- 3 garlic cloves, minced

- 1 onion, finely chopped

- 1 package whole wheat or bean pasta of your choice

- 4 tablespoons olive oil Salt and black pepper, to taste

- ¼ cup basil, cut into strips

- ¾ cup chicken broth, low-sodium

Directions:

1. Cook pasta as directed over pack; rinse and set aside. Get medium saucepan, add oil then warm up over medium heat.

Add onion, garlic and stir-cook until become translucent and fragrant for 3 minutes.

2. Add shrimp, black pepper (ground) and salt; stir-cook for 3 minutes until shrimps are opaque. Add broth and simmer for 2-3 more minutes. Add pasta in serving plates; add shrimp mixture over; serve warm with basil on top.

Nutrition:

605 Calories

17g Fat

53g Carbohydrates

19g Protein

28. Sweet and Sour Salmon

Preparation Time: 10 minutes

Cooking Time: 5 minutes

Servings: 2

Ingredients:

- 4 (8-ounce) salmon filets

- 1/2 cup balsamic vinegar

- 1 tablespoon honey

- Black pepper and salt, to taste

- 1 tablespoon olive oil

Directions:

1. Combine honey and vinegar. Combine to mix well with each other.

2. Season fish fillets with the black pepper (ground) and sea salt; brush with honey glaze. Take a medium saucepan or skillet, add oil. Heat over medium heat. Add salmon fillets and stir-

cook until medium rare in center and lightly browned for 3-4 minutes per side. Serve warm.

Nutrition:

481 Calories

16g Fat

24g Carbohydrates

1.5g Protein

29. Citrus-Baked Fish

Preparation Time: 10 minutes

Cooking Time: 5 minutes

Servings: 2

Ingredients:

- ¼ teaspoon kosher or sea salt

- 1 tablespoon extra-virgin olive oil

- 1 tablespoon orange juice

- 4 (4-ounce) tilapia fillets, with or without skin

- ¼ cup chopped red onion

- 1 avocado, pitted, skinned, and sliced

Directions:

1. Take a baking dish of 9-inch; add olive oil, orange juice, and salt. Combine well. Add fish fillets and coat well. Add onions over fish fillets.

2. Cover with a plastic wrap. Microwave for 3 minutes until fish is cooked well and easy to flake. Serve warm with sliced avocado on top.

Nutrition:

231 Calories

9g Fat

8g Carbohydrates

2.5g Protein

Fruit and Dessert Recipe

30. Chocolate Ganache

Preparation time: 10 minutes

Cooking Time: 16 minutes

Servings: 2

Ingredients

- 9 ounces bittersweet chocolate, chopped

- 1 cup heavy cream

- 1 tablespoon dark rum (optional)

Directions:

1. Situate chocolate in a medium bowl. Cook cream in a small saucepan over medium heat.

2. Bring to a boil. When the cream has reached a boiling point, pour the chopped chocolate over it and beat until smooth. Stir the rum if desired.

3. Allow the ganache to cool slightly before you pour it on a cake. Begin in the middle of the cake and work outside. For a fluffy icing or chocolate filling, let it cool until thick and beat with a whisk until light and fluffy.

Nutrition:

142 calories

10.8g fat

1.4g protein

31. Chocolate Covered Strawberries

Preparation Time: 15 minutes

Cooking Time: 0 minute

Servings: 2

Ingredients

- 16 ounces milk chocolate chips

- 2 tablespoons shortening

- 1-pound fresh strawberries with leaves

Directions:

1. In a bain-marie, melt chocolate and shortening, occasionally stirring until smooth. Pierce the tops of the strawberries with toothpicks and immerse them in the chocolate mixture.

2. Turn the strawberries and put the toothpick in Styrofoam so that the chocolate cools.

Nutrition: 115 calories 7.3g fat 1.4g protein

32. Strawberry Angel Food Dessert

Preparation Time: 15 minutes

Cooking Time: 0 minutes

Servings: 2

Ingredients

- 1 angel cake (10 inches)

- 2 packages of softened cream cheese

- 1 cup of white sugar

- 1 container (8 oz.) of frozen fluff, thawed

- 1 liter of fresh strawberries, sliced

- 1 jar of strawberry icing

Directions:

1. Crumble the cake in a 9 x 13-inch dish.

2. Beat the cream cheese and sugar in a medium bowl until the mixture is light and fluffy. Stir in the whipped topping. Crush

the cake with your hands, and spread the cream cheese mixture over the cake.

3. Combine the strawberries and the frosting in a bowl until the strawberries are well covered. Spread over the layer of cream cheese. Cool until ready to serve.

Nutrition:

261 calories

11g fat

3.2g protein

33. Fruit Pizza

Preparation Time: 30 minutes Cooking Time: 0 minute

Servings: 2

Ingredients

- 1 (18-oz) package sugar cookie dough

- 1 (8-oz) package cream cheese, softened

- 1 (8-oz) frozen filling, defrosted

- 2 cups of freshly cut strawberries

- 1/2 cup of white sugar

- 1 pinch of salt

- 1 tablespoon corn flour

- 2 tablespoons lemon juice

- 1/2 cup orange juice

- 1/4 cup water

- 1/2 teaspoon orange zest

Directions:

1. Ready oven to 175 ° C Slice the cookie dough then place it on a greased pizza pan. Press the dough flat into the mold. Bake for 10 to 12 minutes. Let cool.

2. Soften the cream cheese in a large bowl and then stir in the whipped topping. Spread over the cooled crust.

3. Start with strawberries cut in half. Situate in a circle around the outer edge. Continue with the fruit of your choice by going to the center. If you use bananas, immerse them in lemon juice. Then make a sauce with a spoon on the fruit.

4. Combine sugar, salt, corn flour, orange juice, lemon juice, and water in a pan. Boil and stir over medium heat. Boil for 1 or 2 minutes until thick. Remove from heat and add the grated orange zest. Place on the fruit.

5. Allow to cool for two hours, cut into quarters, and serve.

Nutrition:

535 calories 30g fat 5.5g protein

34. Bananas Foster

Preparation Time: 5 minutes

Cooking Time: 6 minutes

Servings: 2

Ingredients

- 2/3 cup dark brown sugar

- 1/4 cup butter

- 3 1/2 tablespoons rum

- 1 1/2 teaspoons vanilla extract

- 1/2 teaspoon of ground cinnamon

- 3 bananas, peeled and cut lengthwise and broad

- 1/4 cup coarsely chopped nuts vanilla ice cream

Directions:

1. Melt the butter in a deep-frying pan over medium heat. Stir in sugar, rum, vanilla, and cinnamon.

2. When the mixture starts to bubble, place the bananas and nuts in the pan. Bake until the bananas are hot, 1 to 2 minutes. Serve immediately with vanilla ice cream.

Nutrition:

534 calories

23.8g fat

4.6g protein

35. Cranberry Orange Cookies

Preparation Time: 20 minutes Cooking Time: 16 minutes

Servings: 2

Ingredients

- 1 cup of soft butter 1 cup of white sugar

- 1/2 cup brown sugar 1 egg

- 1 teaspoon grated orange peel

- 2 tablespoons orange juice

- 2 1/2 cups flour

- 1/2 teaspoon baking powder

- 1/2 teaspoon salt

- 2 cups chopped cranberries

- 1/2 cup chopped walnuts (optional)

Icing:

- 1/2 teaspoon grated orange peel

- 3 tablespoons orange juice

- 1 ½ cup confectioner's sugar

Directions:

1. Preheat the oven to 190 ° C.

2. Blend butter, white sugar, and brown sugar. Beat the egg until everything is well mixed. Mix 1 teaspoon of orange zest and 2 tablespoons of orange juice. Mix the flour, baking powder, and salt; stir in the orange mixture.

3. Mix the cranberries and, if used, the nuts until well distributed. Place the dough with a spoon on ungreased baking trays.

4. Bake in the preheated oven for 12 to 14 minutes. Cool on racks.

5. In a small bowl, mix icing ingredients. Spread over cooled cookies.

Nutrition:

110 calories 4.8g fat 1.1 g protein

36. Key Lime Pie

Preparation time: 15 minutes

Cooking Time: 8 minutes

Servings: 2

Ingredients

- 1 (9-inch) prepared graham cracker crust

- 3 cups of sweetened condensed milk

- 1/2 cup sour cream

- 3/4 cup lime juice

- 1 tablespoon grated lime zest

Directions:

1. Prepare oven to 175 ° C

2. Combine the condensed milk, sour cream, lime juice, and lime zest in a medium bowl. Mix well and transfer into the graham cracker crust.

3. Bake in the preheated oven for 5 to 8 minutes

4. Cool the cake well before serving. Decorate with lime slices and whipped cream if desired.

Nutrition:

553 calories

20.5g fat

10.9g protein

37. Rhubarb Strawberry Crunch

Preparation time: 15 minutes

Cooking Time: 45 minutes

Servings: 2

Ingredients

- 1 cup of white sugar

- 3 tablespoons all-purpose flour

- 3 cups of fresh strawberries, sliced

- 3 cups of rhubarb, cut into cubes

- 1 1/2 cup flour

- 1 cup packed brown sugar

- 1 cup butter

- 1 cup oatmeal

Directions:

1. Preheat the oven to 190 ° C.

2. Incorporate white sugar, 3 tablespoons flour, strawberries and rhubarb in a large bowl. Place the mixture in a 9 x 13-inch baking dish.

3. Mix 1 1/2 cups of flour, brown sugar, butter, and oats until a crumbly texture is obtained. You may want to use a blender for this. Crumble the mixture of rhubarb and strawberry.

4. Bake for 45 minutes.

Nutrition:

253 calories

10.8g fat

2.3g protein

Poultry

38. Chicken and Olives

Preparation Time: 10 minutes

Cooking Time: 15 minutes

Servings: 2

Ingredients:

- 4 chicken breasts, skinless and boneless

- 2 tablespoons garlic, minced

- 1 tablespoon oregano, dried

- Salt and black pepper to the taste

- 2 tablespoons olive oil

- ½ cup chicken stock

- Juice of 1 lemon

- 1 cup red onion, chopped

- 1 and ½ cups tomatoes, cubed

- ¼ cup green olives, pitted and sliced

- A handful parsley, chopped

Directions:

1. Heat up a pan w/ the oil over medium-high heat, add the chicken, garlic, salt and pepper and brown for 2 minutes on each side.

2. Add the rest of the ingredients, toss, bring the mix to a simmer and cook over medium heat for 13 minutes.

3. Divide the mix between plates and serve.

Nutrition:

Calories 135,

Fat 5.8,

Fiber 3.4,

Carbs 12.1,

Protein 9.6

39. Chicken Bake

Preparation: 10 minutes **Cooking Time:** 30 minutes **Servings: 2**

Ingredients:

- 1 and ½ pounds chicken thighs, skinless, boneless and cubed

- 2 garlic cloves, minced

- 1 tablespoon oregano, chopped

- 2 tablespoons olive oil

- 1 tablespoon red wine vinegar

- ½ cup canned artichokes, drained and chopped

- 1 red onion, sliced

- 1-pound whole wheat fusilli pasta, cooked

- ½ cup canned white beans, drained and rinsed

- ½ cup parsley, chopped

- 1 cup mozzarella, shredded

- Salt and black pepper to the taste

Directions:

1. Heat up a pan with half of the oil over medium-high heat, add the meat and brown for 5 minutes.

2. Grease a baking pan with the rest of the oil, add the browned chicken, and the rest of the ingredients except the pasta and the mozzarella.

3. Spread the pasta all over and toss gently.

4. Now, sprinkle the mozzarella on top and bake at 425 degrees F for 25 minutes.

5. Divide the bake between plates and serve.

Nutrition:

Calories 195,

Fat 5.8,

Fiber 3.4,

Carbs 12.1,

Protein 11.6

Sauces and Dressings

40. Lemon Sauce

Preparation Time: 15 minutes Cooking Time: 15 minutes

Servings: 2

Size/ Portion: 0.3 g

Ingredients:

- 2/3 cup lime juice

- 3 tablespoon extra-virgin olive oil

- 1/4 cup diced scallions

- 3 tablespoons fresh dill

- 1/4 cup shallots, minced

- 1 tablespoon crushed garlic

- 1/2 teaspoon black pepper, fresh ground

Directions:

1. If using canned limes, use lime juice. Combine with oil and lime juice, along with the herbs, in a mixing bowl.

2. Combine all ingredients in a sauce pan. Simmer over medium-high heat.

3. Pour the sauce over the fish and vegetables mixture.

Nutrition:

229 Calories

20g Fat

3.5g Protein

12g Carbohydrates

7 Days Meal Plan

Days	Breakfast	Snacks	Salads and Sides
1	Berry Breakfast Smoothie	Cucumber Sandwich Bites	Balsamic Asparagus
2	Mediterranean Omelet	Yogurt Dip	Lime Cucumber Mix
3	Hearty Berry Breakfast Oats	Tomato Bruschetta	Walnuts Cucumber Mix
4	Garden Scramble	Olives and Cheese Stuffed Tomatoes	Cheesy Beet Salad
5	Summer Day Fruit Salad	Pepper Tapenade	Rosemary Beets
6	Egg, Pancetta, and Spinach Benedict	Coriander Falafel	Squash and Tomatoes Mix
7	Peach Sunrise Smoothie	Chickpeas and Red Pepper Hummus	Balsamic Eggplant Mix

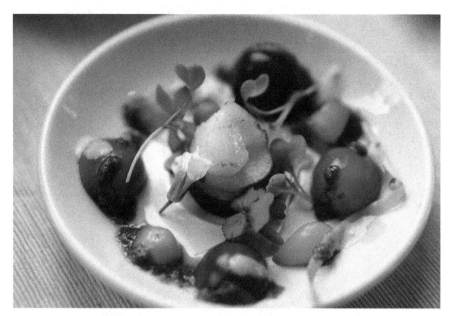

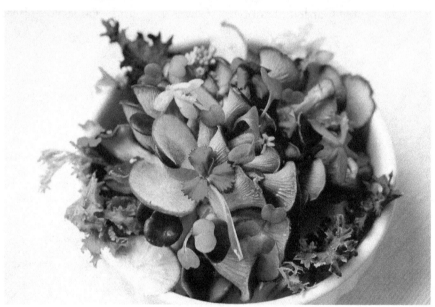

Conclusion

If you're used to consuming fast food, red and processed meats, candy, white flour, sugar, and alcohol, converting to new and whole foods can be difficult.

If you eat mostly unhealthy foods, the risk of cancer, heart disease, high blood pressure, cholesterol, depression, inflammation, low immunity, and other health problems increases dramatically.

This diet will cleanse your blood, enhance your mood and fitness, raise your immunity, and reduce your risk of diseases like type 2 diabetes, breast and colon cancer, and Alzheimer's disease.

Even depression and anxiety have been linked to food preferences, according to studies. Fresh foods grown in the sun have a much better chance of improving your mood.

One of the best things about the Mediterranean diet is that it doesn't need you to be a master chef to cook your meals. You can still make easy and delicious meals with the right ingredients that don't take hours in the kitchen.

Prepare your weekly meal schedule, shop for groceries, and eat just the right foods. You'll have more stamina, your cognitive functions and memory will increase, and you'll never feel bloated again.

The most critical aspect of this diet for people who want to lose weight is to maintain a positive attitude. This is a safe way of life that involves paying attention to what you eat, spending more time with your loved ones, and increasing your physical activity. When you've lost weight, you'll be able to hold it off by just consuming your favorite foods. This diet is incredibly simple to adopt because it does not feel like a diet. Since you'll stick to your Mediterranean menu, there won't be any yo-yo impact. This diet is an excellent way for you to break your bad eating habits and eliminate your junk food cravings. Some foods should be consumed regularly and foods that should be consumed only once in a while.

Recipes decode the Mediterranean Diet Pyramid's principles, transforming it's "less meat, more vegetables" approach into complex, strong one-dish suppers that take the guesswork out of changing partitions and different dishes.

Finally, what matters is that you feel satisfied, happy, and comfortable in your own skin.

In a matter of days, the Mediterranean diet will transform your appearance. It will help you lose weight by improving your physical diet, metabolism, and overall health.

CPSIA information can be obtained
at www.ICGtesting.com
Printed in the USA
LVHW080036050621
689455LV00020B/1209